HEALING YOURSELF WITH WATER

Full details of hydropathic techniques for a variety
of ailments, all of which can be carried out in the
home. Also explains how these water applications
should be used to maintain health and prevent
disease.

HEALING YOURSELF WITH WATER

How You Can Use Hydrotherapy
for Gaining and Maintaining Health

by

J. RUSSELL SNEDDON N.D.

NATURE'S WAY

THORSONS PUBLISHERS LIMITED
Wellingborough, Northamptonshire

First published as *About the Water Cure* in
1965 and twice reprinted
This Edition completely revised and reset 1977

ISBN 0 7225 0309 1

Filmset by
Specialised Offset Services Limited, Liverpool
and printed by
Weatherby Woolnough Limited, Wellingborough, Northants

CONTENTS

INTRODUCTION

Using water to gain and maintain health is a very old cure and it is really difficult to determine when it actually originated but it is known that Hippocrates, the Father of Medicine, spoke about its effectiveness.

About 1800, however, Vincenz Priessnitz, a Silesian farmer's son, noted for his intelligence and excellent powers of observation, became interested in the reactions of sick animals. He found that in the main these animals did not eat during their sickness and tried to get to streams and rivers to bathe in the running water.

Some time later, Priessnitz became involved in an accident, suffering a leg injury which proved beyond medical skill. Then he remembered how sick animals behaved in like trouble and evolved a method of water treatment which in time brought his leg back to normal use. From this point onwards he gained a reputation as a healer by water and he gradually built an establishment which could deal with one thousand patients at a time.

Priessnitz used Sitz baths, full and half baths and compresses, and even today the methods used in our health homes and by practitioners in private practice vary very little from those advised by this pioneer of water treatment, although the theory of the treatment is now more understandable.

It is very interesting to note that about this time Johannes Schroth, also destined to become a great healer, was born in a small village near the birthplace of Priessnitz. Schroth was the originator of the cold compress treatment, used largely in nature cure practice of the present day, and he also taught the benefits of the dehydrated diet which is still practised in this country.

After Schroth came Sebastian Kneipp who became the parish priest of Worishofen, Bavaria. Kneipp was a weakling and brought himself to health by water applications. He set up a water treatment establishment in Bavaria and wrote many articles and books on this form of treatment.

Priessnitz, Schroth and Kneipp all understood that the healing power of water actually depended on the body's reaction to the application and this was the secret of their great success, although it must be stated that towards the end of his career Kneipp began to incorporate certain herbs and other substances in his treatment but basically he still worked on reaction.

Since Kneipp many people have practised the water cure, but very few of them had the personality of the pioneers and they were largely unknown outside their own area. For a time hydropathic institutions in Europe and Britain flourished but the fact that few of them survived is evidence that their treatment departed from the first principles.

Certain health resorts still claim to cure by water, but these have mainly become commercialized and the water is medicated or contains sulphur or other minerals which is supposed to have healing qualities. The methods practised are not those of true hydrotherapy and these practitioners have given in to public belief, namely, that something supposed to be medicated will have a greater effect.

We are now a comfort-loving people and the

term 'Water Cure' conjures up a picture of a very sick person being dipped in medicated water or being bashfully subjected to a powerful jet of water directed at some diseased part of his anatomy. Very naturally the person in sub-standard health turns to some easier and seemingly more civilized method of cure. Granted it is possible for a person to take the water and feel soothed and relaxed but these efforts are gradually weakening. The only real benefit follows when the rather rigorous treatments are followed to a conclusion.

It must be stressed that the methods outlined in this book are not wholly for people who are ailing. Water cure is ideal for preventing disease getting a hold in the body, and if practised in health will do much to retain that desired state. Due to modern living, disease is always ready to enter our bodies, very often without symptoms, and it can penetrate our weakest organs and make some headway with the disintegration of our second line of defence before symptoms make their appearance.

We do not suddenly become ill, and water treatment, practised in conjunction with diet, exercise and correct thinking, forms the perfect defence against this unseen attack. It does so by stimulation of the skin and circulation and by forcing elimination from the deeper organs.

For example, let us study the quick cold Sitz or hip bath. If this bath was practised regularly, say once or twice weekly, the number of cases of womb cysts and tumours would rapidly drop and many surgical operations with resultant misery would be avoided.

The health-giving properties of water are really only appreciated by nature cure practitioners, who advise this cure regularly. This does not make their treatment any easier because most patients need some convincing of the validity of the argument, but the earnest practitioner does not shrink from such difficulties, and as a result many wonderful cures have been wrought. At the same time, it is appreciated that certain people do not react to water applications, indeed, certain types do not react to them at all, a fact mentioned in many homoeopathic books where the study of people's mental characteristics is a feature. In such cases very easy water applications are advised, usually some form of compressing.

Ill-health changes very little although the symptoms vary from time to time, and if the water cure is practised according to the principles of the pioneers we have an excellent method of preventing it and increasing the inherent power of the body towards healing.

In this book the most suitable water treatments for home use are explained with a guide to their application in the treatment of the common ailments.

CHAPTER ONE

THE SKIN

Although there are internal applications in hydro-therapy the skin is the organ most frequently used for the reactions and some knowledge of this tissue is necessary to conduct the treatment successfully.

The skin is composed of several layers and contains nerves, arterial lymph and venous vessels, sweat glands, fat glands, hair and hair roots. It is a complex tissue largely abused and neglected in our modern way of life. It works in conjunction with the other eliminating organs, but in itself has great capacity for the removal of internal impurities, and many people remain alive even when they are very sick as the result of a very healthy skin.

In normal health the active skin eliminates about two pints of impurity daily. This is greatly increased in fever when the skin acts as a control of the internal temperatures. It is also increased in highly emotional persons when a clamminess of the skin shows how the impurities are being eliminated. The perspiration which follows intense physical activity is usually the sign of an active skin and has given rise to the advice: 'For health your skin should perspire at least once daily.'

In peak condition the skin should be fairly dry and easily lifted from the underlying tissues very much like that of a healthy dog. Although seemingly dry it should retain a certain amount of oil and surface moisture. Very dry scaly skin is a sign of ill-health.

During the normal course of the life of a skin cell it is formed in the deeper layers and, as its capacity for work falls, it is moved to the surface of the body. This means that the actual skin we touch is composed of millions of dead cells which are rubbed away by the friction of our clothes. If these dead cells become sticky and adhere longer than normal, the skin when lifted between the fingers exceeds the thickness of one eighth of an inch. Then the functions, especially the eliminative ones, are greatly reduced. So the skin should be fairly dry and should feel thin and pliable when grasped between the fingers. This evenness of thickness should be fairly distributed throughout the body and it is one of the tests for areas of unhealthy skin. A thick skin is an unhealthy one.

A very important point is that our skins should be white or pink and should burn fairly easily in strong sunlight, making careful sunbathing a necessity so that we receive great benefit from this form of bathing. 'Browning' of the skin is only a sign of the skin cells' effort at protection against the strong rays of the sun. It is not so health-giving as a slight skin redness which is allowed to disappear before another exposure.

Although the whole of the skin acts as an eliminating organ, there are certain areas which have a greatly increased eliminative function. These are the armpits, groins, between the legs and the feet. In water treatment these are the parts which should always be kept in good tone particularly the feet, and many people have a poor skin tone in their body but very active glands in the skin of their feet.

So hydropathic reactions depend very much on

the vitality of the person undergoing this cure and particularly on the activity of the skin. This means that very often the primary treatment is directed at getting a loose and fairly dry but thin skin, and achieving this desirable state may be quite difficult and months may pass practising initial skin care before the desired water reaction is obtained for more general health purposes.

INITIAL SKIN TONING

The question of underwear is always important and the best plan for the young and vigorous is to wear very light underwear; if the cold is severe a heavier jacket or coat should be worn. A feeling that it is slightly cold always keeps the skin active, and if this is practised in youth it is likely that the skin will remain in health until well into middle age.

In the weak, middle-aged and elderly, the problem is not so easily solved. Most people feel the need for warm underwear, especially in a variable winter climate. Usually the best plan is to wear a light extra garment next to the skin (string garments are excellent). This allows the skin to breathe and tends to get rid of the layers of moisture which are nearly always present when wool is worn next to the skin. The next thing to do is to practise skin care until it is found that the heavier woollen garment can be discarded in the summer and not replaced during the next winter.

THE FRICTION RUB

Dry and thick skins can be brought back to tone by careful friction rubbing. This is best done on rising and before retiring and should be performed in a warm bathroom so that there is little feeling of chill. Start with the scalp. Press the tips of the fingers of both hands into the scalp and rub vigorously. Gradually work down the body ... the neck, shoulder and arms, chest (use a folded rough towel for the back), abdomen, hips, thighs, legs (avoid any varicosity), and finish with the feet.

If the skin is very thick this sort of friction should be carried out each day for a fortnight, and then a friction glove or a fairly strong nail brush should be used instead of the fingers. This is naturally rougher treatment, but by this time it will leave the skin red and glowing and there will be quite a feeling of well-being after the treatment. Do this night and morning, but after the morning treatment have the friction rub and then, dipping the fingers in cold water, lightly rub the body over and finish with a brisk towelling.

Depending on the condition of the skin, and it must be remembered that very few of us ever pay real attention to it other than for cleanliness, the brush friction and finger-tip cold rubs should be continued for a week or two when finally the brisk cold rub down should complete the preparatory skin treatment.

The best way to have a cold rub down is to fill the bath with a few inches of warm water and then, standing in this, take a very large sponge dipped in cold water until saturated, and starting at the neck work right down the body really rubbing the water into the skin. Puffing and blowing – and yelling, if desired – make the exercise more beneficial because it calls the breathing apparatus into play. Finish with a friction rub with the fingers and then a rough towel or flesh glove and dress quickly to retain the heat reaction. Afterwards you will feel vital and your skin will be able to take its share of elimination.

COLD SHOWER

Many people taking up water cure do not like the cold rub down and prefer the cold shower using the apparatus in which the spray is fixed above the head. This is a very good method for even a weak person, but it should not be practised until the skin has been thinned by the friction and brush rubs.

Using a warm (not hot) shower, play the water on the chest and back and then turn it to cold and do the chest and finally the back, allowing the water to play on the back of the neck and run down the spine. A quick friction rub and brisk towelling and the treatment is over within a few minutes and the body feels refreshed.

COLD BATH

This is the bath for the young, vigorous, healthy person. Cold water is filled to a depth of about ten inches, the hips are lowered into the bath and the water is splashed over the chest. The person then rises and runs in the cold water for a few seconds. A brisk rub down and a wonderful feeling of warmth and vigour permeates the body. This type of bath sends the blood racing. It empties a lot of inner reservoirs and gets a flow through the body which cannot be so well achieved in any other fashion, but as has been stated, it is only for the young and vigorous.

These then are the first steps to hydrotherapy, and all are aimed at getting eliminative action through a dry, thin and elastic skin. They are the first essential to the successful practice of hydrotherapy, and they are explained at the beginning of this book to enable the reader to practice them as he continues to study the more complicated treatments.

CHAPTER TWO

EFFECT OF WATER APPLICATIONS

The pioneers of water treatment soon discovered that it was the secondary reaction to the immersions and sprays which wrought the healings, and true hydrotherapy is still based on these findings, although it must be remembered that their treatment was much more heroic than ours of the present day and that it is likely that their patients were of a sterner mould. To fully understand what is implied we must give a little thought to the method employed by the body to deal with what is, after all, mainly a skin irritant. The following findings are based on the reactions of a healthy skin.

HOT APPLICATIONS

When heat is applied to the skin the nearby arteries dilate, the blood flows and more blood is pushed into the enlarged arteries causing redness and congestion. If the heat is still applied then the blood is more or less locked under the heat and perspiration breaks on the surface of the skin. In a poor skin action this sweating does not take place and then hot applications can be definitely harmful. Let us consider when heat can be applied with advantage.

Chilling. Often we appear to be in perfect health and then, without warning or even without any apparent reason, we suffer from very cold feet. The natural thing to do is to have a hot foot bath and this is quiet sensible and an allowable measure, because very cold feet can bring down the blood

temperature ever so slightly and can result in a
bladder or kidney chill or a bout of haemorrhoids.
So get the feet warm as quickly as possible and
often chilling can be aborted, especially if the
person retires to bed and gets a full night's rest.

Again, when the body is chilled after a soaking
or some form of exposure, a warm bath is an
excellent measure. Here, however, we are dealing
with a very large surface and the tendency,
because it is so comfortable and relaxing, is to
have the bath too hot. Here is an excellent guide.
Have the bath fairly warm but come out whenever
the slightest moisture can be felt on the brow. This
is the sign that the congestion of the enlarged
arteries is getting concentrated, and harm and
even chilliness can result after this bath. If
possible, go straight to bed after a warm bath, but
if this is unsuitable then have a quick cold sponge
down to close the pores. Always finish with a cold
application.

Tension. Many people speak of the relaxing
effects of a hot bath but the best results in this
condition are obtained from a neutral bath, that
is, a just warm bath actually near body
temperature. This bath really soothes the nerves
but does not damage the arteries by prolonged
congestion. Such a bath should last about ten to
twenty minutes, continually adding a little hot
water to keep the temperature just above chilling.
The neutral bath is ideal for all nervous
conditions.

Relief of Pain. The foregoing hot applications are
excellent for the special purposes mentioned and
now we come to the relief of pain, which is one of
the common purposes of hot applications. Hot
bags or poultices, hot water bottles, heat lamps
are the methods commonly used, and here a

warning must be given because wrongly used these can be dangerous.

Heat applied to the skin to relieve pain works in two ways.

1. The sensory nerves underneath the part become tired out and the burning sensation is not conveyed to the brain and tissue destruction can take place.
2. The heat acts as a counter-irritant to the pain beneath and no cure is being wrought.

This means that all hot applications are dangerous, especially so in the following conditions.

(a) In elderly people there is great danger of destroying tissue because the sensory sensation in the brain is not registering the degree of heat.
(b) If there is inflammation in the part such as a lung, bronchial tube, inflamed stomach or bowel, appendix, ovary, boil, abscess or carbuncle, etc., then the heat 'draws' the inflammation and can cause rupture of the part with very serious results. Avoid hot applications in these conditions.

There are some hot-water treatments for pain when the trouble is not over a vital organ or a vein, the eyes, ears and certain other important parts of the body, but on the whole this type of application can have dangerous after-effects and the best home treatment method is the alternate hot and cold treatment described in another chapter. Do not take risks without professional advice and it is always advisable to leave a condition alone rather than apply very hot water, packs or any kind of heat without knowing exactly what is happening.

Later in this book detailed advice will be given regarding the safe treatment of the more common conditions.

COLD APPLICATIONS

In hydrotherapy hot water is called 'dead' water and cold is termed 'alive' water. When cold is applied to the skin, the action, much quicker than that instigated by the hot, is to constrict the blood vessels and force the blood deeper into the system. The part becomes white and often a slight shiver of the skin is recorded. If this treatment is prolonged it can have quite serious results, because the skin becomes more and more deprived of blood.

Such treatments are nearly always uncomfortable and, as a result, the application time is always short and then the brain tissues recording a local coldness rapidly send blood from the liver into the circulation and the part affected becomes rapidly supplied with fresh and vigorously coursing blood. This is the reaction wanted in true hydrotherapy.

Hot and cold applications can be applied too long and in both cases the reaction is not beneficial to the person. Time is a great factor in all water treatment. A hot or warm application should never be prolonged because it causes the blood to congest and stagnate. A cold application prolonged causes a kind of surface anaemia and this is just as serious as the hot method. Every water application should be short and the actual duration of the methods about to be outlined will be given.

Reaction to cold varies with the individual. In most cases a short treatment will result in a good flow of blood but there are certain people who do not react to any water application and especially a cold one. Dr Lindlhar, the father of nature cure, stressed this point and he maintained that blue-eyed people could stand the cold water and that brown-eyed people were not good patients for this type of treatment.

In many years of practice I have not found that this rule really holds good, because people with good density brown eyes appear to be excellent patients for hydrotherapy. Dr Lindlhar also studied homoeopathy and in this method of treatment one of the important mental character-istics looked for in patients is whether they shun cold in any form. These people do not react to water application and this should never be forced upon them.

In all water treatment the vitality of the patient is most important. The weakly will not react at first and once an application has not achieved the desired reaction it should be discontinued. It may be tried again at a later date. It is also important that treatment should not be given when the stomach is loaded or when the person is tired and mentally or emotionally upset. Even in a very strong person the mildest treatment should be used as a guide to the patient's reaction and if this is good then a gradual increase in severity is indicated.

CHAPTER THREE

CONDITIONS REQUIRING CARE IN HYDROTHERAPY

It is difficult to generalise in this form of treatment because the vitality of the patient is the most important point and even very elderly people take cold baths and receive great benefit from them. There are certain indications which preclude the use of baths, however, and the following come within this category:

Old Age. In old age there is usually some hardening of the arteries with consequent rise in blood-pressure. Sudden immersions or other cold applications in such cases can be too vigorous and the judicious use of cold compressing is the best water treatment. In prostate trouble in elderly men the tepid Sitz bath should be used instead of the cold one, at least until it is obvious that a good reaction will be obtained.

Infancy. Infants do not generate much heat and so the coldest water ever used in their treatment should be tepid. Cold compresses, however, are suitable if muslin or very thin linen composes the compress. Hot-water bags should be placed alongside the infant during this treatment unless there is a very high fever.

Fatigue and Exhaustion. When a person is exhausted the body is demanding rest and the vitality is usually not sufficient to generate the heat required after the cold application. It is very dangerous to have a cold bath, even of very short duration, in these circumstances, and severe chilling is the most likely result. A neutral bath may be helpful at this time but it is very likely that complete rest and relaxation is the best treatment.

Certain nervous ailments, such as asthma, leave the sufferer nervously exhausted and here again the cold application is usually not indicated. To get relief from the asthmatical spasm, however, alternate hot and cold packs may be used even when the patient is really tired. Again, in asthma the stomach and lungs are both deranged and a narrow waist compress (cold) can be used with advantage provided the patient is kept warm with the aid of hot water bottles.

Heart Trouble. Mild cold water administration such as compressing can be used to strengthen the heart, but hot baths and hot applications are definitely contra-indicated, also deep cold hip baths.

Rheumatism. The rheumatic patient generally shuns the use of cold water as a therapeutic agent believing that any such treatment will make the rheumatism very much worse. In such cases, however, the hot baths and other applications of heat are usually only of temporary benefit and the real cure comes within the compass of the cold application, which is never harmful when correctly and intelligently applied.

Start with some form of heat treatment building up vitality with cold rubs and small cold compresses until finally a major cold application can be taken with benefit. It is appreciated that not every rheumatic sufferer feels that dampness in any form is harmful, but here the same building towards major cold water treatment is still advisable.

Chest Cases. In asthma, heart trouble, high blood-pressure, thrombosis of the coronary arteries, avoid the use of a chest spray which can have a too stimulating effect on tissues already weakened.

High Blood-pressure. Usually warm and hot applications such as Sitz and mild steam baths lower the pressure as a secondary reaction and can be used with care, but cold applications must only be taken under professional supervision.

KIDNEY IRRITATION
Determination of the right amount of fluid intake

necessary for the health of a person is always difficult because it varies with the individual. The trained practitioner can tell from skin examination when such intake is too much or too little and give advice accordingly. It is also possible after a short study of a patient's reactions to tell from the skin if a patient has taken fluid which is irritating the kidneys. This requires experience but it can be done with a very low percentage of error and it points out that kidney distress is mirrored on the skin.

A famous physician once said that we should drink eight pints of fluid daily to flush out the kidneys, and from that day to this many people have flushed their kidneys until these organs have become diseased.

What happens when we take a large quantity of liquid in any one day? First of all, it is very likely that we weaken the digestive juices of the mouth, stomach and small bowel causing a kind of indigestion. Next, the large amount of water irritates the bowel through a laxative action which works for a time and then the tube becomes too flaccid, loses tone and constipation results. Finally, this fluid comes to the kidneys and they are forced to work all day and often during the night, causing discomfort all round. In the end we have a tired and worn-out person with worn-out kidneys.

Other writers tell us to drink only when naturally thirsty. What is natural thirst? Supposing a person partakes of a meal having a fish and meat course liberally sprinkled with seasoning and with added salt, is the thirst which follows a natural one? Again, is the thirst which comes after a cabinet bath, be it of steam or vapour, or even after a Turkish bath, a natural one? No! These are unnatural thirsts and should be quenched only with very small quantities of fluid.

The thirst of a fever or after strenuous exercise, or one which arises in very hot climates, are more of the natural varieties and may be quenched rather liberally but only with water, which is the only solvent needed by the body. The best water is that distilled by nature into vegetables and fruits and taken along with the whole substance, because even expressed fruit and vegetable juices have lost some of their balance.

As a guide to the amount of fluid let us consider the following. If swellings of the loose tissues beneath the eyes, in the fatty parts of the abdomen, or in the legs and ankles and feet take place, then too much liquid is being introduced and is not being dealt with by a tired heart and kidneys. A much more dry diet is necessary in such conditions. If there is indigestion, even of the mildest degree, then I would advise the taking of dry meals and a suitable liquid between meals. Dry meals, very thoroughly masticated, can work wonders in most digestive difficulties.

What are suitable liquids? First of all, take your liquid in solid form, that is, in fresh fruit and vegetables. If thirst is experienced take water, and actually there is never any need to drink anything else. However, most people of unnatural palate feel they need a more interesting fluid and small quantities of yeast extract drinks, cereal coffee, vegetable soup and milk may be taken between meals. China tea and home ground coffee may be taken on limited occasions but they have very little health value and are definitely more destructive than otherwise.

CHAPTER FOUR

METHODS OF APPLICATION

Now follows a description of the various water applications which, providing the skin care already outlined has been followed, can be used to maintain and regain health.

They are all uncomplicated but require determination until the benefits become apparent. The rewards are great because water, properly applied, is the greatest of all healing agents. Used as described they are never suppressive.

When used to maintain health a general scheme should be arranged suiting your age and physique and this should be carried out at regular intervals. If you have a personal illness, then choose the water treatments which are advised at the end of this book, arrange them in a scheme and practise them carefully until a positive change is obtained, when the treatment can be reduced in severity.

In professional practice the patient is given a programme of water cure, which naturally varies with each patient, but is along the following lines.

Each day on rising: Have a cold shower, then hand rub, and finally friction rub.

Two mornings weekly: Alternate hot and cold hip bath. Duration ten minutes.

Waist compress: Five nights weekly. Neck compress to be used on three nights, along with waist compress.

The golden rule is to always include some skin treatment in every scheme.

ALTERNATE HOT AND COLD APPLICATIONS

There are various theories why one person should suffer from bronchitis and yet another person, living under practically the same circumstances, should have a disease of the bowels. Each type of practitioner tends to think of a certain cause. The medical man believes that a collection of bacteria in the part causes the difficulty; the surgeon thinks of poor tissue; the osteopath believes that some lesion of the spine has brought about poor circulation, and so on.

Whatever the cause, the body, perceiving that the blood and tissues are becoming overloaded with impurity, seeks to direct this toxic material to a part which is not vital. This may be the scalp and then dandruff results; in the frontal sinuses it is called sinusitis, inflammation of the tonsils is known as tonsilitis, and so we have bronchitis, colitis, leucorrhaea from the womb and vigorous sweating from the feet. When the skin is full of toxins then we have skin disease, boils, abscesses and carbuncles.

It will be appreciated that all these 'dust-bins' have the power of discharge and so the body can, within limits, get rid of its impurity, in an effective though unnatural manner. It will be understood by readers that if the normal organs of elimination with which the body is amply supplied, the kidneys, lungs, bowels and skin, were working well there would be no need for such dust-bins.

The unfortunate point here is that whenever we get a discharge of any kind, instead of wondering what is the real meaning behind it, we tend to stop it with some medication, get it cut out, or suppress the body's attempts at cleansing and it is then that the dust-bins can really become overloaded and often a more vital organ becomes engorged.

Hydrotherapy by its very nature works mainly on the skin and it follows that this eliminating organ or tissue soon becomes more and more efficient. This is one of the reasons why it is claimed to prevent ill-health. If, however, a 'dust-bin' becomes overloaded and severe inflammation results, which water treatment is suitable? Here we must follow one of the golden rules ... 'When in doubt use alternate hot and cold.'

These applications are 'safe.' They act very much like an artificial pump in that they stimulate blood flow and venous and lymphatic drainage, and when applied to the congested 'dust-bin' they rapidly bring about a reduction in inflammation.

The hot application, used so frequently in home treatment, is always a dangerous one when applied to any type of inflammation and if used over a vital organ, such as the lung, kidney, appendix or bowel, can often bring about an increase in inflammation with consequent rupture and serious complication. So we have the rule ... 'Never apply a hot application over a vital organ.' In hydrotherapy hot water or steam are always dangerous and must be used generally and never locally, except on the skin and then never over an internal organ.

Hot and Cold Showers. To invigorate the skin, especially in a weakly person, a shower is ideal. Use the hot shower on the back and then the front of the body trying to get a comfortable force. Do this for two minutes and then have a short cold shower of thirty seconds, and then again use the hot shower for two minutes.

The percussion effect of the shower is valuable in addition to the thermal changes and this type of treatment can be taken for ten minutes always starting with the hot and finishing with the cold application. After this rub the skin vigorously with a rough towel, flesh gloves or fairly hard brush or, best of all, with the hands until the skin is dry, red and glowing.

This treatment is tonic but not so effective in gaining tone as the quick cold shower by itself. Alternate hot and cold showers are more health-giving than the hot bath and, if necessary, the first application of the hot water can be made over the body which has already been soaped for cleansing purposes. For skin health it is essential that all soap should be washed away, and this is especially true in scalp treatment where soap can have a very irritating effect. In professional treatment strong jets of water from a hose are used to get deep acting percussion effects but these are not suitable for home treatment.

The Falling Shower. This is one of the best applications for nervous people. Actually the greatest benefit follows when only cold water is used but alternate hot and cold is often advised at the beginning of the treatment. Usually the rose is removed from the ordinary vertical shower and then the water drops vertically without spreading or having real force ... The patient stands directly below the shower, allowing the water to strike just at the base of the neck and run down the spine. Again use two minutes hot and a half minute cold alternatively, starting with the hot and finishing with the cold. After the nerves have become strengthened, stop the hot application and use a quick cold falling spray.

Limbs. The knees, ankles and feet are parts which are frequently benefited by alternate hot and cold administrations. A small rubber spray fitted to both taps is the most suitable means of applying this treatment, but placing the damaged knee or leg under the hot and cold water tap in turn and letting the water run down the leg is also effective. When treating the feet, two basins, one with hot water and the other with water from the cold tap, are all the apparatus required.

Packs. Pack treatment is used for local application over the injured or inflamed part. They are composed of pieces of flannel of several thicknesses because this material retains the heat. Soak the first pack in very hot water, wring out and apply, keeping it on the part from two to three minutes and then apply the cold pack soaked in ordinary tap water (not ice cold) for one minute. The duration of this treatment is usually from ten to twenty minutes depending on the strength of the patient and the part being treated. The pack should always be folded in such a way that it completely covers the area under treatment to get the full benefit.

Sitz or Hip Baths. These alternate hot and cold immersions supply an excellent means of stimulating the organs of the lower abdomen and pelvis. They are fully described in the chapter on Sitz baths.

CHAPTER FIVE

SITZ AND CABINET BATHS

We come now to one of the best hydropathic measures, the Sizt or hip bath. Not so many years ago, specially designed and movable hip baths were to be found in many homes but these were used for economic cleansing purposes.

Nowadays the designed hip bath is very

expensive and, indeed, it is difficult to obtain one in this country, most of them being imported from Germany. Ideally two baths are used, to enable the patient to get alternate hot and cold hip baths, and these are frequently used in the hydropathic and nature cure institutions.

Without this special bath most of us have to do as best we can with the ordinary bath, the smaller ones being most suitable because in this application the feet should not be in the water.

The Cold Sitz Bath. Using the ordinary bath, fill it at least half full of cold water between the temperature of 50° to 60° F (10° to 15° C) and immerse the hips so deeply that the water comes up to the umbilicus. Put the feet on a towel at the end of the bath.

Duration of this bath: Should be short, two or three minutes, and never longer than five minutes.

Headache. Certain people find this bath very beneficial but are troubled with a headache afterwards. This can be prevented by having the feet in hot water before or during the bath, or by placing a cold towel round the head for a bath of long duration and a hot towel for a short duration bath. At the end of the bath do a 'hundred up' (stationary running) in a few inches of cold water or spray cold water on the soles of the feet.

Effects of the Cold Sitz Bath: The heart beat is slowed and becomes fully and stronger. Arterial tension is increased and there is a great flow of fresh blood through the parts which have been immersed.

Nervous System. The nervous system of all pelvic and lower abdominal organs is greatly stimulated. The lower spinal nerves, especially those around the coccyx, are rapidly retoned.

Incontinence. A quick shallow cold Sitz bath is

excellent for children who suffer from incontinence of urine of a physical nature. Can be used daily or on alternate days, but the duration should never exceed a few minutes.

Weakened Sexual Power. A deep 60° to 70° F (15° to 21°C) Sitz bath of about five to ten minutes. duration is excellent for this trouble. In women it should not be used during the period times and where there is any pus formation.

Prolonged Menstrual Flow. Give a deep cold Sitz of a few minutes' duration from the fifth day after menstruation should cease.

Slipped Pelvis. Where pelvic and hip muscles are weak and hip slips out of place easily, this is the ideal treatment.

Persistent Diarrhoea. Start with fairly warm water (about 85°F, 30°C) and gradually reduce to 60°F (15° C). Do this for two days and then afterwards keep reducing the water temperature until it reaches 50° F (10° C) in five minutes. Keep rubbing the immersed parts all the time. Duration of this treatment should never be more than five minutes.

Biliousness and Liver Troubles. Cold Sitz of two minutes' duration is very tonic.

Constipation. When this condition is chronic a cold Sitz bath ten inches deep and of two minutes' duration will be found a most excellent treatment.

WHEN COLD SITZ BATHS ARE NOT ADVISED

Womb bleeding: In such circumstances professional advice should be sought.

Inflammation with pus formation in any part of the abdomen and pelvis: An examination is necessary to determine the cause.

Colic and muscular spasms of the abdomen and

pelvis: Again, examination is necessary to discover the cause of the trouble before water applications are commenced.

The Hot Sitz Bath. In this bath the water should be really hot (about 108° F 42° C) and the duration of the bath should be approximately five minutes.

It is useful in: Bladder or Kidney Chill; General Body Chill (when full bath is not suitable); Excellent for General Nervous Tension.

A very hot Sitz bath, practically as hot as can be borne, is an excellent treatment for confirmed alcoholics and people who have been taking drugs. The finish to such a bath (in these cases) should be application of a towel wrung out in cold water and applied down the spine, or a more spartan treatment is a bucket of cold water poured down the back. These methods are very effective in delirium tremens.

In hydropathic institutions and in health homes the alternate hot and cold Sitz baths are used very frequently with very tonic results. At home the ordinary bath may be used for the hot Sitz and a large tin, rubber or plastic basin used for the cold.

The hot water should be kept at a temperature in the region of 104° F (40° C) and the cold water straight from the tap. Two minutes hot and a slightly shorter period in the cold bath, alternately for six to ten immersions is the normal duration of this treatment, always finishing with the cold application.

Conditions which indicate the need for hot and cold Sitz bath:

1. Strain of hip muscles.
2. Painful nervous contraction round lower spine.

3. Painful or delayed menstruation.
4. Haemorrhoids.
5. Neuralgia of ovary.
6. Inflammation around genitals.
7. For sexual weakness.
8. General toning.
9. Recurring hip slip.

STEAM BATH

This bath is taken in a box or tent-like structure which may be movable and easily erected in a bathroom. The patient sits on a stool with the head and neck outside the bath and steam is generated by a small boiler. Usually the heat is raised fairly slowly and this bath can therefore be made quite relaxing and soothing, and the attendant can arrange the temperature to suit the patient. Frequently this bath is too prolonged, because little benefit from the viewpoint of the output of skin impurity, is gained after the initial sweating. After this the heat only removes excessive moisture in the body, and from this angle it is a very successful treatment in modern slimming establishments.

Afterwards the patient is placed on a table and the skin is rubbed with a mixture of salt and water or by the hands dipped occasionally in cold water. Rest, sunray and a little exercise complete what is really a very soothing and cleaning treatment and this accounts for much of its popularity.

SAUNA BATH

In its proper setting the Sauna bath is excellent for cleansing the uppermost tissues of the body. The bathers sit or lie in a room in which a fire has heated large stones to a very high temperature. The attendant then throws water on these stones and the resultant steam heats the atmosphere and brings about a profuse sweating on the part of the bathers.

This sweating is carried on until the bather begins to feel exhausted, when he or she is subjected to a cold bath, shower and a rub down and then rest. In certain countries the final cooling down consists of going out naked into the snow and diving into a half frozen lake. This rather heroic treatment calls for a good skin action and great vitality.

Baths arranged on these lines can be obtained in large cities in Britain and are to be recommended, but the sweating should not be prolonged.

CHAPTER SIX

THE DOUCHE AND THE ENEMA

The perineum or floor of the pelvis is an area of soft and lightly muscled tissue forming the part behind the generative organs and in front of the anus.

It is an area of great importance because if tone is lost here, then the tendency is for the rectum, bladder and womb to be, first of all, displaced and then to drop downwards (called prolapse), and this in turn causes all sorts of miserable conditions. Lack of tone in these organs spreads rapidly and the bowel, urinary tracts are frequently involved. This means that when treating loss of tone in the perineal muscles we must also treat the rectum, bladder and womb. Most physicians employ exercises to regain tone and, in the surgical sphere, the dropped organs are stitched up.

The perineal muscles can be over-exercised. These muscles require a certain amount of relaxation and this is especially necessary in childbirth. Too much exercise can tighten them too much as seen in the case of women gymnasts, ballet dancers and the like. These women often have a very painful time at childbirth due to their perineal muscles being too tight. After surgical stitching of prolapse light exercise and water treatments are indicated.

So in lack of tone of the pelvic organs, haemorrhoids, prolapsed rectum, displaced uterus, bladder troubles, enlarged prostate and general falling of the contents of the pelvis, in weakened sexual powers and lack of power to evacuate the bowel contents, the perineal douche can be used with great success. If graded exercises, under the care of a competent practitioner are also practised, then most of these conditions can be helped and many of them completely cured.

Before describing how the douche is given there are certain rules which must be followed.

1. The bladder and rectum must be emptied before the douche is used. Do not, however, strain at the stool unless there is some desire on the part of the bowel to move.
2. The douche should not be used during the normal duration of menstruation. It can be used as described after the menstruation has ceased.
3. All protrusions should be reduced before the douche is used. A protruding rectum or womb can usually be easily replaced, although bathing with hot water may be required to get this done satisfactorily. In the

case of haemorrhoids, hot soapy water bathing should gradually reduce the tension of the rectal muscle and allow the piles to be reinserted. Failing this, give a prolonged hot perineal douche to get the same effect. It it is impossible to reduce the pile mass then do not use the cold perineal douche.

Essentially the spray consists of a jet of water, at varying pressure, playing against the floor of the pelvis behind the generative organs. Usually the patient is sitting and the spray is directed upwards. In most houses on the Continent the bidet, a spraying apparatus, is to be found in the bathroom, and this is a useful aid which takes up very little space. It is based on the same design as the low set lavatory pan but has a spray in the centre and two knobs which control the flow of hot and cold water. It is ideal for all forms of perineal douching and is valuable in the treatment of many troubles of women. A simple do-it-yourself apparatus can be built for this purpose along the following lines:

A piece of wood of length to extend from one side of the bath to the other and some ten inches broad and one inch thick has a four inch hole cut in the centre of its length. Beneath this is fixed a pipe with a three-eighth inch opening, the end of the pipe being a few inches beneath the board. The water pipe is fixed to the other end of this pipe and, if possible, this could be connected to both the hot and cold tap to allow varying sprays to be used.

The treatment is conducted in a warm bathroom and a few inches of hot water in the bath keep the feet warm. Sitting in such a fashion to get the jet midway between the generative organs and the anus, the jet is gently turned on and gradually increased in intensity until it just stings but does not cause real pain. The duration of the application should never exceed two minutes. In people who are very much below par the first jet can be modified to luke warm water and then to a final sharp short spray of cold water.

In haemorrhoids or womb prolapse the treatment is varied slightly. First of all, a cold low pressure spray is directed at the rectal opening or at the vagina. This can be kept until slightly painful and then the spray should be directed at the mid perineal area for general tonic effect. Remember that protrusions should be reduced before this treatment.

COMMON TREATMENTS

Atonic Condition of the Bladder. Start with luke warm spray and work on to a quick cold application. Keep the feet warm during the treatment. Spray behind the generative organs.

Impotency and Sexual Troubles. Do not use the hot spray. Start with a very short cold spray and then work up to the two minute spray.

Constipation (due to lack of power in the rectal area). Use a fairly strong pressure hot spray for two minutes, and cold one for half a minute. Continue alternately for ten minutes and finish with a quick cold spray.

Haemorrhoids (piles). One minute on perineal centre part and one minute on rectal area using strong cold spray.

Depression and Introspection. The perineal spray or douche affects the whole body and in people suffering from the conditions this treatment tones up the nervous system and gives them a much more buoyant outlook. Use the cold douche on

alternate nights for a fortnight, making the
duration about one minute.

Prolonged Menstruation. Many women are troubled
with prolonged menstruation, lasting many days
over the normal of four or five days. The perineal
douche can be curative in this condition. Use hot
water in the bath or basin to keep the feet warm or
put a cold compress round the head to prevent
headache. Apply the cold perineal douche from
the fifth day of the period making the application a
short one of about one minute. Continue, if need
be, daily until the flow stops. Cold compressing is
also advised, using the waist compress high above
the umbilicus.

Prostate Trouble. In middle-aged and elderly men
the Tee compress (see p. 45) should first of all be
used to get tone back to the prostate gland. After a
week or two of this treatment a lukewarm perineal
douche should be taken for about two minutes,
and then a very quick cold perineal douche of
about one minute's duration. This simple
treatment can be most effective in this annoying
condition and has often prevented the need for
surgery. Always remember that the bladder must
be emptied as completely as possible before this
douche.

WHEN THE PERINEAL DOUCHE IS NOT ADVISED

1. Severe abdominal inflammation. In such
   cases a cold compress is the safe treatment
   and professional advice should be sought.
2. Colic or muscular spasms in the abdomen.
   Again, the cold compress may be worn.
3. During normal menstruation.
4. Near bedtime. Douching can disturb normal
   sleep.

THE ENEMA

Many people suffering from a sluggish bowel use the warm water enema whenever they feel internally clogged. This is not good practice because, in addition to making the bowel lazy by not forcing it to work itself, the enema removes internal secretions and oils and dries the bowel in an unnatural manner.

Everyone has a natural bowel rhythm according to physical make-up and emotional stability. This rhythm may be a bowel movement after each meal; it may be a bowel movement once daily, or the bowel may move naturally every second or even third day, and so on. The rhythm varies with the individual and once it is established it must be accepted as part and parcel of the person's make-up. If, however, it is obvious that the bowel is not clearing itself, shown by symptoms such as headache, furred tongue, general lassitude and a greasy and unhealthy skin, then the rhythm has been established on a poor diet and an unhealthy way of life.

To force this bowel by laxatives or enemas is the wrong approach. Here a careful diet, well chosen with regard to eliminative foods and a system of exercise, especially of the abdominal muscles, will bring about a change in the bowel rhythm, and this will soon become an established and healthy bowel movement. This does not mean that a very active bowel is a healthy one. Many, many people who have reached the century have had a very slow bowel rhythm, say a movement every third or fourth day, but they were not actually constipated because there are no signs of impurity within the bloodstream. The enema should, therefore, be only used as an emergency measure in the following conditions:

1. After surgical operations, not affecting the bowel or stomach. In these cases, the giving of an anaesthetic often causes a partial paralysis of the bowel and a very chronic constipation can then ensue. A warm water enema can bring great relief and stimulate recovery.

2. Excessive flatulence after a severe nervous shock. An enema can then give tremendous relief but it should be used sparingly.

3. During very high fever when the sufferer is fasting but the high temperature seems to be drying the bowel juice.

4. When the body has been poisoned.

5. During fasting. Often when fasting is used as a health measure the accumulated toxins within the body and bowel cause a very coated tongue, headache, general nausea and weakness. A warm water enema each night of the fast will usually speed the cure.

THE TECHNIQUE

There are several forms of enema but those most suitable for home use are the syringe and the can. The latter is best and consists of a can, which holds several pints of water suspended several feet above the bath. From this runs a long rubber tube with a valve and a nozzle at the end. The can is filled with water slightly warmed (comfortable to the elbow dipped in it), and with or without the addition of a small amount of soap.

First of all, make sure all the air is removed from the tube by allowing some water to flow and, lying on the left side, the nozzle of the enema, slightly smeared with vaseline, is introduced into the rectum and the valve opened to allow a little water to flow into the anal canal. This may cause a little pain at first and the flow should be stopped until this ceases.

After this gradually allow the contents of the can to flow into the bowel. Once the flow ceases, lie on the back with the knees up and then on the right side, and finally back to the left. Retain the water within the bowel until it becomes really uncomfortable. In many cases the first enema is not too successful, but if another one is taken immediately afterwards the bowel contents are easily released. Children in high fever should be given a half pint enema in an effort to control the temperature.

THE HIGH ENEMA

In this type the water is forced much farther up the bowel and some ten pints of water are used, but here it is wise to get this treatment under professional care, otherwise it is possible to do harm. Many people feel this type of apparatus holds the key to their health and are very disappointed when they are unable to get such treatment. Although unwilling to condemn this attitude entirely, it would appear that better results could be obtained by ensuring intestinal cleanliness by attention to diet which really holds the key to inner health.

CHAPTER SEVEN

TYPES OF COMPRESSES

The pioneers of water cure, mainly through a study of animal reaction, discovered that moist heat was very healing. They also found that the most suitable way of getting this heat reaction was through the application of a compress or pack to the skin after these had been soaked in cold water. The size and thickness of the pack or compress varied with the part being treated.

The cold moist compress works in two ways:

1. After the initial application comes the reaction and fresh blood flows rapidly to the part, supplying food and removing impurity. It will be appreciated that if the blood-stream is pure and healthy a better effect is obtained, so water cure and good dietetics work hand in hand.

2. The moist compress also results in the expressing of impurities through the skin. These are naturally gathered into the compress, which in turn means that the cloths after application often contain very poisonous substances and should be boiled thoroughly before being used again.

Throughout the years as compressing was developed, a technique was evolved based on the following:

THE WAIST OR MAIN COMPRESS

It was found that if a compress was applied on the waist area to cover the kidneys and main abdominal organs, the assimilation of food was greatly aided, elimination was increased and this was one of the best treatments for the sluggish bowel. Again, this waist compress was found to have a stimulating effect on the kidneys, increasing the output of nearly solid impurities.

This compress is arranged as follows: First of all, obtain a piece of thin linen between six and ten inches broad (it can even be broader), and of a length to go once round the waist and overlap only two inches for fastening with tapes or safety pins.

This is soaked in cold water, wrung out firmly, and applied directly to the waist.

By itself this linen would take a long time to heat, therefore it is covered with one or two layers of warm woollen material which should completely overlap the linen, being fixed with safety pins. This compress may be worn at any time, but in chronic illness it is usual to apply it when retiring, keeping it on all night.

It is necessary that the compress heats up within ten to fifteen minutes, and this is easily checked by inserting the fingers between the linen and the skin. If the heat does not arise then take the compress off, rub the skin with a rough towel and try again next night.

There is always the chance of the compress not heating, many factors causing this such as tiredness, nervousness, emotional upset and so on. Very often the compress will heat for a few weeks on end and then suddenly it fails to get the desired reaction.

As has been stated in chronic cases the waist compress is worn at night and removed in the morning, and it is usual to apply it for five nights weekly and then to allow two nights to pass without compressing. In acute cases the waist compress can be worn all the time until some control over the trouble is gained.

It will be occasionally found that the skin under the part covered with the compress becomes discoloured. This need not cause any alarm, being a sign that the compress is bringing out impurities, and after two or three nights without compressing the discolouration will fade and then this treatment can be resumed.

THE NECK COMPRESS
In addition to the waist compress other parts of the body can be treated at the same time. These smaller compresses are called 'local' and they can be used over any part of the body. The neck compress is very frequently applied because here two main nerves of the body are near the surface, and can easily be impinged or irritated by tensions of the neck muscles. This compress consists of a piece of linen some three inches broad and of a length to go once round the neck and overlap one inch for fastening. This linen is soaked in cold water, wrung out and applied firmly to the neck and covered with flannel or woollen material.

In the same way, the foot, knee, hand, elbow or any muscular part needing attention can be compressed. Certain parts, due to the contours of the body, make compressing difficult. Take, for instance, the shoulder. Here a local compress is difficult to apply and so a thin singlet is used, the shoulder of which is soaked in cold water, wrung out, worn and covered with some warm material. The same technique is applied when the chest or back has to be compressed, but it must always be remembered that local compressing must be accompanied by a waist compress. Using both compresses ensures a good eliminative cleansing through the blood stream, whereas local compressing may do harm by bringing impurities to the spot.

In certain cases of high fever the whole body is enveloped in a body compress or pack. This is a piece of thin linen, soaked and thoroughly wrung out. This is laid on the bed and the patient is then covered with it. On top are placed plenty of blankets and use can be made of hot water bottles to get the heat to develop quickly. This is a rather heroic treatment and is usually conducted under the care of a practitioner, but it is excellent in cases of high fever in a patient who is still very vital.

THE TEE COMPRESS

In this arrangement a strip of linen, three inches broad, is attached to the back of the waist compress. This strip goes between the legs and is again attached to the front of the compress. This tee compress is used in certain specific conditions.

CHAPTER EIGHT

TREATMENTS FOR SPECIFIC AILMENTS

Abscess. If this occurs in a part removed from a vital organ the main treatment is compressing, using a waist compress and a local one which covers the abscess and, in most cases, this will be enough to reduce the inflammation and disperse the forming abscess. If, after some time, the condition does not improve then use alternate hot and cold packs several times in one day, and then again use the compresses.

In most cases this will stop the formation of the condition, but if it continues to form, then I believe in letting the skin rupture itself and not following the usual advice of applying hot packs. If the skin ruptures itself the healing is usually excellent without scar formation, especially if after rupture, local and main compresses are used to get the part thoroughly drained. After healing, oil the scar each night with warm olive oil and soon all trace of it will disappear.

If the abscess occurs in the neck, use only a neck

and main compress and, if possible, take only fruit
and fruit juice to clear the drainage systems. It is
not a good plan to apply heat over any glandular
part such as the neck, armpit or groin.

Amenorrhoea. This means the absence of
menstrual flow. Between the normal period times
use hot and cold hip baths, a perineal douche
(cold) and a Tee compress applied five nights
weekly. Tone up the general system with cold rubs
and, if possible, obtain sun baths. Compressing
and all water treatment should be stopped at the
times when menstruation should appear and
commenced again five days later.

Aphonia (hoarseness and loss of voice). In this
condition the vocal chords are either chilled or
overstrained. Apply hot and cold packs to the
throat for fifteen minutes and do this several times
daily. Steam the face and head at night, adding a
little Friar's Balsam to the water. Neck and waist
compress should be worn at any convenient time
until recovery is full and then twice weekly for a
month. If the person overstrains his voice in his
occupation, then occasional neck and waist
compresses will be of great benefit in preventing a
recurrence.

Arthritis. Treatment depends greatly on the
position of the trouble. In the hand, wrist and
elbow, alternate hot and cold packs accompanied
by local and main compressing are indicated. In
the spine the falling shower, alternate hot and cold
shower, spinal and waist compress. In the lower
spine the hot and cold hip baths are best
accompanied by a waist compress and
occasionally by a cold perineal spray. If in the
legs, hot and cold hip baths or hot and cold
showers to the affected parts and alternate hot and
cold foot baths will prove of great help. Remember

that hot and cold applications are the safe means of reducing pain and stimulating circulation.

Anaemia. If this condition is severe, reaction to water treatment may be difficult to obtain. The waist compress, using very thin linen, is the best starting point and this should gradually be increased in depth until the compress stretches from the umbilicus to the armpits. This compressing of the chest and ribs often stimulates the production of blood. When some progress has been made the alternate hot and cold perineal shower can be used, and skin care using the friction rubbing first of all, and then working to the cold rub, will bring a retoning. Too copious menstrual periods or bleeding haemorrhoids should be treated by appropriate measures.

Angina. This trouble can be alleviated by water cure. The neck compress is invaluable but it is wise to commence with a narrow waist compress and use this for several nights before adding the neck one. This compress eases the tension on the vagus nerve which has a control over the heart action and has been known to completely cure the condition, although I think that other health measures are still indicated. If the person is overweight then recourse to dieting is necessary and hot and cold hip baths and mild sweating baths will then be of benefit. Hot and cold alternate packs to the front of the chest are often helpful in relieving the actual spasm of the attack.

Asthma. In the acute attack alternate hot and cold packs, applied to the front or back of the chest (the results vary with the individual), are usually of the greatest value. At other times apply waist and neck compresses and, when the person is well again, continue with this system of compresses for at least three months. Alternate hot and cold hip

baths and cold perineal douching is needed when
the asthma is of digestive origin.

Atrophy. Wasting of muscle can arise from
several causes but alternate hot and cold
applications, choosing the method most suitable,
are most useful in retaining tone. Waist and local
compressing of the affected area should be
continued if a reaction is obtained, but often this is
difficult in serious cases. Note that if nerve tissue is
damaged it may be impossible for the person to
tell when the application is too hot and care must
be exercised.

Backache. This is a symptom of many diseases,
but when associated with a muscular condition it
will be found that alternate hot and cold hip baths
(of about fifteen minutes' duration) nightly for a
week will usually remove the ache. If the condition
has been allowed to become chronic or there is a
continual strain on the back muscles through
occupation, then a cold compress around the part,
applied five nights a week, will keep the muscle in
much better tone. The whole body cold sponge
down and friction rub should be practised daily.
Very often the pelvis 'slips' when muscles are weak
and one leg becomes longer than the other. This
requires correction from a practitioner and the
cold or alternate hot and cold hip baths help
greatly.

Baldness. If not of nervous origin, men troubled
in this way should dip their heads in cold water
each morning, and once or twice weekly should
give the head a hot and cold head dip, always
finishing with the cold application and drying the
hair vigorously with the fingers. In severe cases a
local compress of linen can be cut and shaped to fit
the scalp. This is worn nightly along with a waist
compress.

When the trouble is of nervous origin (Alopecia) the alternate hot and cold hip baths are indicated along with a cold perineal douche and neck and waist compresses. Arrange a scheme along the following lines: Hot and cold hip baths once weekly. Perineal douche twice weekly. Hot and cold head baths or sprays twice weekly. Neck and waist compresses five nights weekly. This treatment has been very effective in many cases.

Bell's Paralysis. A paralysis of the muscles of the face on one or both sides causing inability to close the eye, smile or show the teeth. When due to cold, apply hot packs to side of face in front of the ear for about twenty minutes, and then cover the affected part with a warm woollen cloth. This hot pack treatment can be applied several times daily. The patient should also have a warm bath of some twenty minutes' duration and again the hot packs should be used on the face. Rub warm olive oil into the face before retiring. Immediate treatment after a chill is best and it should be concentrated for the first few days until some nervous control is gained. After this wear a neck and waist compress each night.

Bladder Inflammations. Many people know that if their feet become cold or wet they will suffer from inflammation of the bladder. In most cases this can be avoided by immediately having a hot hip bath which is very effective and can be taken in the ordinary bath as described. Failing this, bathe the feet in hot water for twenty minutes, always keeping up the heat, and retire to a heated bed. When there is chronic inflammation of a varying nature, such as cystitis, the best application is the alternate hot and cold perineal douche accompanied by an occasional hot hip bath, working towards the alternate hot and cold hip bath once the bladder has gained muscular control. The amount and kind of fluid taken with the diet is also important and requires study.

Bile (sluggish flow). Very often people are told after X-ray examination that they have a sluggish bile flow. Diet plays a big part in this condition, but the use of alternate hot and cold packs over the gall bladder area, that is, below the lower right ribs, will stimulate the gall bladder action. A large waist compress should be worn covering this area, five nights each week.

Blood-pressure (Low) In this condition there is general tiredness and lack of tone in the blood vessels. The alternate hot and cold perineal douche is excellent at the start of water treatment and this should be carried out five nights weekly. After this, have a quick cold hip bath of a few seconds' duration as a tonic treatment. Continue to wear the cold compress until the blood-pressure is normal again.

Blood-pressure (High) Alternate hot and cold hip baths twice weekly with a prolonged neutral bath on other two occasions and a waist compress each night to stimulate kidney function makes an excellent treatment in high blood-pressure. Short duration steam cabinet baths also reduce blood-pressure.

Boils. A local and a waist compress is the best water treatment, and this often reduces the boil without further treatment. If the boil bursts wear a small piece of wet linen (over the wound changing it frequently) and do this until all pus is expressed. Hot applications often complicate matters.

Breast Disorders *Abscess*: Treat as described for abscess with breast and main compress. Keep breast supported and warm.

Enlarged: Due to fat formation. Spray breasts

with alternate hot and cold water and practise exercises which raise the breasts and bring about drainage.

Mastitis: Spray the breast with hot and cold water and compress the breast, using also the main waist compress for chronic mastitis. Milk is not recommended in the diet of a person suffering from this condition.

Bronchitis. In the acute condition the greatest benefit is achieved by using alternate hot and cold packs over the painful congested parts of the chest, and doing this frequently, say every three hours for about fifteen minutes. This treatment is also useful for occasional application in the chronic form of bronchitis, using it some three times weekly, and also wearing a compress over the congested area and one on the waist at the same time. In bronchitis it is also necessary to pay great attention to skin care and, whenever possible such a sufferer should be having cold rubs or cold sprays morning and again at night to get the skin working as an eliminator of the great amount of impurity which is always present in this condition.

Burns. A clean sheet of linen, soaked in cold tea, applied to the wound and kept damp by another piece of wet linen applied over the first, which is never allowed to become dry, is one of the best ways of treating a burn. The first piece of linen is never removed but is cut away as the skin is renewed. Scar formation is greatly reduced by this simple method of treating even severe burns. After healing apply hot olive oil to the part nightly.

Bursitis. This can occur in any joint and means inflammation of a bursa, a protective arrangement. Immediately it is discovered apply hot and cold alternately, using a spray or packs, always finishing with the cold application. Then apply a cold compress binding this fairly tightly. Local compressing is allowed for several days, but if it is obvious that the treatment will be prolonged, then wear a waist compress at the same time as the local cold one.

Chilblains. Cold is the best application and, if the circulation is good enough, a quick cold foot bath is the treatment. Failing this, spray the bunion with alternate hot and cold water using some force, and then wear a local compress over the bunion with one on the waist.

Croup. The water treatment for this condition is exactly the same as that described for asthma.

Deafness. When due to catarrh, water treatment can be of great benefit. Internal crackling and spasmodic deafness after or during a cold should be treated by gargling frequently with a full glassful of warm water, and in this particular condition cold water should never be used for gargling. If continual deafness follows then apply hot and cold packs to the area just below the ear on several occasions daily for about ten minutes. At night wear a neck and waist compress. Skin should be stimulated as much as possible using cold sponges and even cold Sitz bath. Continue to gargle with warm water to clear the Eustachian tubes.

Diarrhoea. If the feet become chilled, hot foot baths will often prevent the stomach and bowel from becoming chilled. If the chill results in diarrhoea, a warm bath or, better still, a hot hip bath will often relieve it. If it is long continued and weakening, warmish, not hot, hip baths should be continued over a period. In this condition the cold waist compress is not advised, because there is danger in chilling.

Dropsy. Or hydrops, is swelling of the loose

tissues and, when pressed, this swelling shows an indentation. If it is found in the ankles and feet after a strenuous day's work it usually has no great significance. If it appears without any real reason then it usually means that the heart or the kidneys are not in good tone. In all types of dropsy the dry diet, taking liquid (limited to water, fruit and vegetable juices) between meals and in very limited quantities is the best hydropathic measure.

As the fluid in the tissues is retracted and expelled some extra strain may come on the kidneys and a waist compress every alternate night will be of benefit. If the heart is involved the dry diet, with neck and waist compressing, will prove very helpful. Walking is the best exercise to get the drainage going, and this combined with the above water cure will aid any other help measures.

Dyspepsia. In all cases of indigestion the type of food and when it is taken are very important. Water treatment should be based on waist and neck compressing. The neck compress eases the tension in the muscles of this area and this has a beneficial effect on nerves which control some of the stomach actions. In addition, the waist compress greatly increases the nutrition of the stomach itself, and these compresses have often resulted in a wonderful improvement in cases of weak digestion.

If the stomach is very large and pendulous some falling of the organs will have taken place, and then alternate hot and cold hip baths, with an occasional very short cold hip bath, will do much to retone these muscles. The perineal douche can be used when it is felt that the reaction to hip baths is not strong enough, but always the waist compress should be worn. Where there is prolonged pain in the stomach this compress often has a very soothing effect.

Emphysema. This term means that there has been over-distension of the air cells of the lungs, often resulting in some quite large cavity formation. It will be appreciated that once these cells have lost their shape no real recovery is possible. With general health measures, dieting and breathing, it is possible to get some health back into the lungs and then water cure can be most helpful. The skin care is invaluable here, aided by hip baths to stimulate the bowel and kidneys, and the treatment should be continued, with neck and waist compressing, several nights weekly. When the patient feels much stronger, alternate hot and cold packs to the chest will bring new blood to the lungs.

Empyema. Usually this term is applied to the chest and it means that pus has gathered in the pleural cavities. It will be appreciated that this patient must be far removed from health before this happens, and the condition must always be regarded as serious. Usually drug treatment is applied and here this may be the best in the initial stage and then water treatment can be of the greatest importance in getting drainage.

Many years ago I was called to treat a girl suffering from a very serious attack of this trouble. Surgery had been advised but even this was not supposed to be of much avail. She was placed on a very dry diet, hot and cold compresses were applied frequently to the affected side, and between times she wore a large body compress called the wet sheet. The nurses who were attending the girl watched this treatment with some dismay, but after five days the girl regained strength, came out of her comatose condition, and from that minute slowly came back to health.

She compressed for months afterwards and made a full recovery and to this day she has never had another serious illness. This demonstrated to the medical men and surgeons involved the wonderful healing power of the water cure and diet and, indeed, I have heard that one of them still uses these methods since seeing this wonderful cure.

Fever. One famous physician has stated: 'Give me a fever and I can cure any ailment,' meaning that such upsets were actually nature's healing efforts and that if allowed to carry out this aim, then the body would be healthier afterwards. Modern methods of treatment tend to reduce the temperature, quickly controlling the fever and often, it would appear, stopping the cleansing.

Water treatment actually presents the best way of controlling fever, that is, keeping it within bounds and yet allowing the internal upset to be beneficial. In even a mild fever the body should be sponged frequently with slightly warmish soapy water to remove the poisons which come out in the perspiration, finishing with a quick coldish rub down and a change of pyjamas. If the fever rises then a waist compress should be worn and changed whenever it becomes dry. Usually this will control the fever, but the compress can always be enlarged until it reaches from the armpit to the waist.

If such a size of compress is necessary, it means that the sufferer is in a poor state of health and the compress will 'draw' away a great deal of impurity and will prove a life saver. Always boil the compress after the application. In fever of any severity the compress is just worn under the pyjamas, no other covering being necessary. In such cases sleep is vital and a sleeping patient should never be awakened to change a compress. In severe fevers the enema should be used to clean the bowel.

Fractures. Naturally in any fracture an X-ray examination is necessary to ensure that the bones have been correctly aligned and it is also usual practice to keep the part in place with plaster. Very little water treatment can be done until these bandages are removed. Then apply alternate hot and cold packs to the part twice daily for about twenty minutes. This speeds the healing and after this the best treatment is the cold spray used occasionally or, if suitable, a cold immersion. At night a waist and local compress should be worn.

These compresses can be worn long after the fracture has completely healed, because they greatly improve the blood supply and drainage to the new formed bone and to the muscles and ligaments which often are severely hurt when the injury takes place. This means that compressing for two months after the injury occurred will do nothing but good, and the complications of fractures will thus be avoided.

Remember that there will be a slight swelling of the healed area for a year or two afterwards due to laying down of new calcium deposits on the bone. This swelling can never be removed by compressing nor is it wise to attempt its removal.

Gall Bladder (sluggish action). Many of us have a slow action gall bladder, mainly due to overtiredness because most of us eat too many fats or complicated fatty mixes. The best treatment for the sluggish gall bladder is alternate hot and cold hip baths twice weekly, to get a general increase in the tonicity of the abdomen. In between times apply hot and cold packs alternately to the part over the gall bladder just below the ribs on the right side or slightly towards the middle of the abdomen. This treatment has a very marked stimulation of bile flow. At night a waist compress will keep the stimulation still effective.

Many people are also troubled with a chokage of the common bile duct lower in the abdomen. This is the duct through which the bile passes on its way to the bowel and this chokage often takes place near the umbilicus, and is shown by tenderness in this area and by constipation and lack of energy. If it is severe, jaundice may even result. It would appear that hot applications would be the most suitable but you must remember that these are always dangerous over the abdomen, and again alternate hot and cold packs over this part with an occasional cold hip bath are best, and often bring a marvellous result.

When a gall stone, formed in the gall bladder, attempts to pass down the narrow tract the patient can suffer a great deal of pain, which seems to radiate from a point just near the lower right ribs. This pain is really a colic and can be very intense. Here a prolonged hot pack will often bring great relief, and this is one condition in which such an application is allowed.

After the pain subsides I am inclined to stop all water treatments and let the patient rest, because it is possible with wrong treatment to stimulate the common bile duct again into action and this can cause a renewal of the pain. In most cases an X-ray examination should be obtained and, if the result is negative, it usually means that the gall bladder contains consolidated bile, and this can be gradually removed by dietetic attention and by using alternate hot and cold packs twice or three times weekly.

Glandular Swellings. There are many reasons why gland swell. Chill, infection of a part draining into the gland, general glandular fever, chokage of the duct draining the gland and other causes can be identified. Water treatment is always tricky because it really depends on the cause of the swelling, and the best and safest plan is to put a small cold pack (always keeping this wet) over the swollen gland and to compress the waist at the same time. This will gradually reduce the swelling.

Goitre. Slight swellings of the thyroid gland occur from time to time, very often during pregnancy and at menstrual times. In most cases, these are of little consequence and local and waist compressing will soon bring the gland back to normal. When the thyroid gland really enlarges and other symptoms, such as pulse and weight variations, appear then a neck and waist compress should be worn six nights weekly, alternate hot and cold hip baths should be taken twice weekly and, whenever possible, an osteopath or naturopath consulted to ensure that there are no spinal lesions of the neck area. Do not submit to surgery or any drastic injection treatment until these water treatments have been tried.

Hay Fever. Experience has proved that this is generally a catarrhal condition and attention to diet is the basic cure. Very often the facial sinuses are choked with this catarrh and hot and cold applications to the forehead and around the base of the nose will often bring rapid relief. A neck and waist compress can be used to continue the treatment. In severe cases, the head steaming bath should be practised. In this a basin is filled with boiling water, adding a little Friar's Balsam. Cover the head with a large towel and, leaning over the basin, let the steam play on the face till perspiration is profuse.

Headache. Naturally many troubles have headaches as a symptom and the water treatment varies considerably.

Congested Headache: Treatment should be directed to the lower part of the body and hot and cold hip baths, bathing the feet in cold water and running for a few minutes in three inches of cold water in the bath will relieve most headaches of this nature.

Sinus Headache: Hot and cold packs alternately to the facial sinus on the forehead and around the base of the nose. Head steaming is also of use.

Neuralgic Headache: In neuralgia, a prolonged hot pack followed after some time with alternate hot and cold packs will bring great relief.

Bilious Headache: Apply hot and cold packs to the liver area and have a quick cold hip bath.

Rheumatic Headache: Coming from neck area ... Prolonged hot application and then alternate hot and cold packs, and finally a waist and neck cold compress.

Hernia. If the hernia is very large, then professional advice should be sought, because there is danger of the bowel become strangulated. Small hernias often respond to water treatment and exercise. A toning system based on the following should be arranged, but first of all lie flat and gently reduce the hernia with finger pressure. Then spray the part with cold water trying to get as much force in the water as possible. After this, have a quick; about thirty seconds, cold hip bath, splashing the water over the hernia, and finally apply a compress in such a way that it covers the hernia and applies a firm pressure. Usually this treatment will retone the muscles and the hernia will disappear, but care must be taken when lifting heavy weights and straining at stool.

Influenza. The dangers of influenza cannot be overstressed and every effort should be made to remove the toxaemia as quickly as possible. Whenever the person feels cold and shivery and generally unwell, a prolonged hot bath is indicated, and when perspiration breaks he or she should be sponged down with warm soapy water, a waist compress applied and they should retire to a heated bed.

If they manage to sleep it is likely that they will feel better on wakening, but if restless and fevered then a fairly large compress should be applied to the waist to bring away poisons, and the body should be sponged with warm soapy water to cleanse the skin. Remember that the linen of the compress should be boiled after each application. In severe attacks with much fever a whole body cold sheet bath can be used, provided the patient achieves a moist heat, and this can be very healing indeed. Care always is necessary to make sure that the compress heats up and when this is achieved then nothing but good will result. Waist compressing should be continued for weeks after the influenza has resolved. The golden rule is keep in bed until really well.

Lactation (poor milk flow). Hot and cold packs applied to the breasts will stimulate the flow of milk when this is scanty. If, after the baby is finished with breast feeding, the breasts are hard and knotty then hot and cold packs applied at regular intervals will do much to clear this condition and this will often prevent serious breast trouble in later life.

Muscles (torn). Muscles are often torn due to excessive effort or as the result of fatigue, and frequently healing is prolonged. Resting the muscle is always the best course, but immediately the trouble has occurred alternate hot and cold sprays or packs applied over the area will speed the healing. During rest the local compress over the tear, accompanied by a waist compress, will also help. During the healing the quick cold spray is of service, because it keeps stimulating the blood flow.

Neuralgia and Neuritis. In both conditions the usual treatment is prolonged heat, but far better results are obtained from alternate hot and cold immersions, compresses or packs. Neuritis is often made worse by hot applications and the cold compress will usually be found to be of greater service.

Ovary. Inflammation of an ovary is characterised by a pain deep on either side of the lower abdomen. It very frequently occurs just before and after the menstrual period. A large compress, cut so that it fits neatly into the part and worn on alternate nights between the normal period times, will often completely cure this trouble. Alternate hot and cold hip baths are also useful. Note that no cold application is advised during the menstrual time, although warm baths may be taken.

Pleurisy. The same treatment as detailed for empyema.

Prolapse (of any of the abdominal organs). In any form of prolapse the quick cold hip bath is really invaluable, and I have known many people get completely cured by regular treatment of this nature, but of course it demands a certain amount of vitality on the part of the patient. Hot and cold alternate hip baths suit the more weakly patient and the wearing of a Tee compress will aid the cure.

Rheumatism. Every kind of rheumatism can be treated by water. In the smaller joints quick cold water immersions or the more easily applied cold sprays are excellent. When the trouble is in the hips alternate hot and cold hip baths will soon restore the circulation and an occasional cold hip bath should be taken. Alternate hot and cold packs can be used in all other conditions where immersions and sprays are not suitable. Local and waist compresses can be used with great success on any part afflicted with rheumatism.

As an eliminative treatment steam and electric cabinet baths of short duration, just long enough to bring out the first perspiration, will do much to lower the amount of impurity in the system and so let healing proceed. Pine baths are also healing but should be taken infrequently because they are weakening to certain people. In every case of rheumatism time must be spent getting the skin into tone, cold water being excellent in this connection.

Skin Disease. Some skin ailments are made worse by water treatments, but generally it will be found that the neutral bath is very soothing to the irritated skin. Again, many skin conditions react well if after a warm (not hot) bath the skin is lathered with a soap containing oil and this lather is allowed to dry on the skin.

Remembering our four main organs of elimination, it follows that when the skin is overworked we must stimulate the others, namely the lungs, bowel and kidneys. The cold waist compress encompasses the bowel and the kidneys and hot and cold packs or sprays over the chest will get the lungs more active, and so these are the basic treatments in any form of skin ailment.

Local irritations of the skin can be treated by

cold compressing (always using a waist compress at the same time). Steam and electric baths are excellent for clearing the skin of any pustular rash.

Sleeplessness. Alternate hot and cold hip baths or even foot baths, followed by a cold waist compress are very effective in any form of sleeplessness. After using compresses for a length of time it will be found that the deepest and most restful sleep follows their use. Many people fall asleep on going to bed but waken in the early hours and cannot get to sleep again, and if this takes place over a lengthy period the health begins to decline. The cure is easy although uncomfortable. A waist compress should be put on when the person wakens during the early hours! If this is done on each occasion then a full night's sleep is experienced in a very short time.

Varicose Veins. It is not possible to completely cure this condition once it is established but the tendency to enlarged veins can often be overcome by giving the legs a quick cold spray each morning and following this with a brisk walk. Hot and cold hip baths aid greatly in reducing congestion of the lower abdomen and a waist and leg compress worn five nights weekly will soon take the tiredness from the veins and reduce the tendency to ulceration.

INDEX